Ways to increase personal attractiveness to other

A guide for mastering the art of lasting impression

Richard S. Willis

Table of contents

Chapter 1:Introduction: Understanding Personal Attractiveness

Personal attractiveness is a multifaceted concept that encompasses various aspects of physical appearance, social skills, confidence, and emotional intelligence. It plays a significant role in how individuals are perceived by others and can influence the quality of their interpersonal relationships, professional success, and overall well-being. In this chapter, we will explore the fundamental components of personal attractiveness and delve into the importance of understanding and cultivating it in our lives.

Physical Appearance

One of the most visible aspects of personal attractiveness is physical appearance. While beauty standards may vary across cultures and societies, there are certain universal qualities that are often associated with attractiveness. These include factors such as facial symmetry, clear skin, healthy hair, and a well-proportioned body. However, it's essential to recognize that beauty is subjective, and attractiveness is not solely determined by external features. Confidence, personality, and charisma also play significant roles in how attractive a person is perceived to be.

Social Skills

Beyond physical appearance, social skills are essential in determining personal attractiveness. Effective communication, active listening, and empathy are crucial components of social competence. People who are skilled in interpersonal interactions can build rapport, establish connections, and make others feel valued and understood. These individuals are often perceived as likable, approachable, and charismatic, qualities that enhance their overall attractiveness.

Confidence

Confidence is another key aspect of personal attractiveness. Individuals who exude confidence are more likely to attract positive attention and admiration from others. Confidence is not about being arrogant or boastful but rather about having a strong sense of self-worth and self-assurance. Confident individuals are comfortable in their own skin, assertive in their actions, and resilient in the face of challenges. Their self-assurance is contagious, drawing others to them and enhancing their overall attractiveness.

Emotional Intelligence

Emotional intelligence, or EQ, refers to the ability to recognize, understand, and manage both our own emotions and the emotions of others. High emotional intelligence is associated with greater interpersonal effectiveness, improved communication skills, and stronger relationships. People with high EQ are adept at navigating social situations, resolving conflicts, and building meaningful connections with others. Their ability to empathize, communicate, and connect emotionally makes them highly attractive individuals.

Understanding personal attractiveness is about recognizing that it extends far beyond physical appearance. While physical attractiveness certainly plays a role, it is just one aspect of a much broader concept. Social skills, confidence, and emotional intelligence are equally important factors In determining personal attractiveness. By cultivating these qualities, individuals can enhance their interpersonal relationships, professional success, and overall quality of life. In the chapters that follow, we will delve deeper into each of these components, exploring practical strategies for developing and maximizing personal attractiveness in various areas of life.

Chapter 2:Enhancing Physical Appearance

Personal appearance plays a significant role in how we are perceived by others and can impact our confidence, self-esteem, and overall attractiveness. While physical attractiveness is subjective and influenced by cultural norms, there are universal practices that can help individuals enhance their appearance and feel more confident in their skin. In this section, we will explore three key aspects of enhancing physical appearance: grooming and personal hygiene, dressing for success, and maintaining fitness and health.

Grooming and Personal Hygiene

Grooming and personal hygiene are essential components of maintaining a polished and presentable appearance. Good grooming habits include regular bathing, skincare, haircare, and grooming of facial hair (if applicable). Proper hygiene practices not only help individuals feel fresh and clean but also contribute to their overall health and well-being. Cleanliness and grooming reflect attention to detail and self-respect, qualities that are attractive to others. Additionally, grooming can boost self-confidence and self-esteem, leading to a more positive self-image.

Dressing for Success

Dressing for success involves selecting clothing that is appropriate, flattering, and aligned with one's personal style and professional environment. The way we dress communicates messages about our personality, professionalism, and attention to detail. Whether it's dressing for a job interview, a business meeting, or a social event, choosing the right attire can make a significant difference in how we are perceived by others.

When selecting clothing, it's essential to consider factors such as fit, color, fabric, and style to create a cohesive and polished look. Dressing well not only enhances our appearance but also boosts our confidence and self-assurance, allowing us to present our best selves to the world.

Fitness and Health

Physical fitness and health are integral components of personal attractiveness. Regular exercise, balanced nutrition, and adequate sleep are essential for maintaining a healthy body and mind. Exercise not only helps individuals achieve and maintain a desirable physique but also releases endorphins, reduces stress, and improves mood and confidence. A nutritious diet provides the body with essential nutrients, fuels energy levels, and promotes overall well-being. Sufficient sleep is crucial for physical and mental recovery, cognitive function, and overall health.

Prioritizing fitness and health not only improves one's physical appearance but also enhances vitality, energy, and attractiveness.

Enhancing physical appearance involves grooming and personal hygiene, dressing for success, and maintaining fitness and health. These practices contribute to a polished and presentable appearance, boost confidence and self-esteem, and positively impact how individuals are perceived by others. By investing time and effort into these areas, individuals can enhance their overall attractiveness and present their best selves to the world.

Chapter 3:Developing Social Skills

Developing Social Skills is an essential aspect of personal and professional growth. Effective communication, active listening, empathy, and emotional intelligence are integral components of this developmental process.

Effective communication

Effective Communication is the cornerstone of successful interactions. It involves conveying messages clearly and concisely, both verbally and nonverbally. Verbal communication encompasses the use of words, tone, and delivery to express ideas and convey emotions effectively. Nonverbal communication, on the other hand, includes body language, facial expressions, and gestures, which often communicate more than words alone.

Mastering both verbal and nonverbal communication is crucial for building strong relationships and fostering mutual understanding.

Active listening

Active Listening is another vital skill in the realm of social development. It goes beyond simply hearing what someone is saying; it involves fully engaging with the speaker, understanding their perspective, and empathizing with their feelings. Active listening techniques such as paraphrasing, summarizing, and asking clarifying questions demonstrate genuine interest and help ensure that the speaker feels heard and valued. By actively listening, individuals can strengthen their relationships, resolve conflicts more effectively, and build trust with others.

Empathy and emotional intelligence

Empathy is the ability to understand and share the feelings of others. It involves putting oneself in another person's shoes and seeing the world from their perspective. Cultivating empathy requires both emotional awareness and compassion. Through active listening and genuine curiosity about others' experiences, individuals can develop a deeper understanding of their emotions and needs. Empathy fosters connection and fosters a sense of belonging, contributing to healthier relationships and a more empathetic society.

The capacity to appreciate anyone on a profound level envelops the capacity to perceive, comprehend, and deal with one's own feelings, as well as the feelings of others It involves self-awareness, self-regulation, social awareness, and relationship management. Self-awareness enables individuals to recognize their emotions and understand how they impact their thoughts and behaviors. Self-regulation involves managing impulses and emotions in constructive ways, even in challenging situations. Social awareness allows individuals to understand the emotions and needs of others, while relationship management involves effectively navigating social interactions and building strong connections.

Developing social skills such as effective communication, active listening, empathy, and emotional intelligence is essential for personal and professional success. By honing these skills, individuals can improve their relationships, enhance their leadership abilities, and contribute positively to their communities. Through practice, self-reflection, and a genuine desire to connect with others, anyone can develop these crucial social skills and thrive in today's interconnected world.

Chapter 4: Cultivating Confidence

1. Cultivating Confidence:

- Confidence is an attractive trait that exudes self-assurance and competence.
- Ways to cultivate confidence include setting and achieving small goals, practicing self-care, and surrounding yourself with supportive people.
- Embracing failure as a learning opportunity can also boost confidence by reinforcing resilience and adaptability.

- Confidence is not about being perfect but about accepting oneself and having faith in one's abilities.

2. *Overcoming Self-Doubt*:

- Self-doubt can hinder personal attractiveness by projecting insecurity and uncertainty.
- Techniques to overcome self-doubt include challenging negative thoughts, practicing self-compassion, and seeking feedback from trusted mentors or friends.
- Building a growth mindset, focusing on personal strengths, and reframing failures as opportunities for growth can help combat self-doubt.
- Accepting imperfections and embracing vulnerability can also foster self-acceptance and reduce self-doubt.

3. *Assertiveness and Self-Assurance*:

- Assertiveness involves confidently expressing one's thoughts, feelings, and needs while respecting the rights of others.
- Developing assertiveness skills includes practicing effective communication, setting boundaries, and advocating for oneself in a respectful manner.
- Cultivating self-assurance can help individuals feel more comfortable asserting themselves in various situations, leading to greater personal attractiveness.
- Assertive individuals are perceived as confident, decisive, and capable, which can enhance their appeal to others.

4. *Positive Body Language:*

- Body language plays a crucial role in communication and can significantly impact how others perceive us.
- Positive body language cues include maintaining eye contact, smiling, standing or sitting upright, and using open gestures.
- Avoiding negative body language signals such as crossed arms, fidgeting, or avoiding eye contact can convey confidence and approachability.
- Practicing mindfulness and being aware of body language can help individuals project confidence and enhance their personal attractiveness.

Incorporating real-life examples, anecdotes, and research findings can further enrich your essay and provide credibility to your arguments. Additionally, discussing the importance of authenticity and genuine self-expression in cultivating personal attractiveness can add depth to your analysis. Remember to conclude with a summary of key points and practical takeaways for readers seeking to enhance their personal attractiveness through confidence, assertiveness, and positive body language.

Chapter 5:Fostering Genuine Connections

In our interconnected world, fostering genuine connections has become an essential skill. Whether in personal or professional settings, the ability to build rapport and establish authenticity in interactions can greatly enhance one's attractiveness to others. This chapter explores strategies for finding common ground, cultivating authenticity, and ultimately, increasing personal appeal through meaningful connections.

Finding Common Ground

One of the most effective ways to build rapport is by finding common ground with others. This involves actively seeking out shared interests, experiences, or values that create a sense of connection. Whether it's a passion for a hobby, a similar life experience, or shared goals, identifying commonalities can lay the foundation for genuine rapport. By demonstrating an understanding and appreciation for what binds us together, individuals can bridge divides and foster deeper connections.

Authenticity in Interactions

Authenticity is critical to building trust and affinity with others. Authentic individuals are genuine, honest, and true to themselves in their interactions. They do not hide behind a facade or try to be someone they are not. Instead, they embrace their strengths and vulnerabilities, allowing others to see them for who they truly are. Authenticity breeds authenticity, and by being genuine in our interactions, we invite others to do the same, creating a more meaningful and fulfilling exchange.

Cultivating Authenticity

Cultivating authenticity requires self-awareness and introspection. It involves identifying our values, beliefs, and passions, and living in alignment with them. This may require vulnerability and courage, as it often means stepping outside of our comfort zones and embracing our imperfections. However, the rewards of authenticity are profound, as it allows us to connect with others on a deeper level and build relationships based on trust and mutual respect.

Practical Strategies for Building Rapport

Building rapport is both an art and a science, requiring empathy, active listening, and genuine interest in others. Practical strategies for building rapport include:

1. **Active Listening**: Listening attentively to others demonstrates respect and fosters understanding. Practice active listening by maintaining eye contact, nodding, and paraphrasing what others say to ensure comprehension.

2. **Empathy**: Empathy is the capacity to comprehend and talk about the thoughts of others. By putting ourselves in someone else's shoes and acknowledging their emotions, we can build rapport and strengthen our connections.

3. **Authentic Communication**: Be honest and transparent in your communication, expressing yourself authentically and openly. Avoid pretending to be someone you're not or hiding behind a mask of politeness.

4. **Finding Common Ground**: Look for shared interests, experiences, or values that create a sense of connection.

Whether it's a mutual love for a hobby or a shared experience, finding common ground can deepen rapport and foster meaningful connections.

5. **Building Trust**: Trust is the foundation of any relationship. Be reliable, consistent, and true to your word to build trust with others. Avoid gossip, deceit, or manipulation, as these erode trust and undermine rapport.

Fostering genuine connections, building rapport, and cultivating authenticity are essential skills for increasing personal attractiveness to others. By finding common ground, embracing authenticity, and practicing practical strategies for building rapport, individuals can forge meaningful connections that enrich their personal and professional lives. Ultimately, it is through genuine connections that we find fulfillment, belonging, and a sense of purpose in our interactions with others.

Chapter 6: Demonstrating Kindness and Empathy

Introduction

In a world often fraught with challenges and complexities, the qualities of kindness and empathy stand out as beacons of light, fostering deeper connections and enhancing personal attractiveness. Acts of kindness and displays of empathy not only benefit those on the receiving end but also contribute to one's own well-being and social standing. This essay explores various ways in which individuals can cultivate and demonstrate kindness and empathy to increase their allure to others.

Acts of Kindness

Kindness, often described as the quality of being friendly, generous, and considerate, manifests in myriad forms, ranging from simple gestures to profound acts of benevolence. One of the most accessible ways to spread kindness is through random acts, such as holding the door open for someone, offering a compliment, or assisting a stranger in need. These seemingly small actions have a ripple effect, creating a positive atmosphere and fostering goodwill within communities.

Beyond spontaneous gestures, deliberate acts of kindness can have a transformative impact on both the giver and the recipient. Volunteering time and resources for charitable causes not only serves those in need but also cultivates a sense of purpose and fulfillment within individuals. Whether it's donating to a food bank, participating in community clean-up efforts, or volunteering at a local shelter, the act of giving back strengthens social bonds and amplifies personal attractiveness.

Showing Empathy and Understanding

Empathy, the ability to understand and share the feelings of others, lies at the heart of meaningful human connection. Cultivating empathy involves actively listening to others without judgment, acknowledging their emotions, and offering support and validation. One way to demonstrate empathy is through compassionate listening, where individuals provide a safe space for others to express their thoughts and feelings without fear of criticism or dismissal.

Empathetic communication goes beyond words, encompassing nonverbal cues such as facial expressions, tone of voice, and body language. By tuning into these subtle signals, individuals can better connect with others on an emotional level, fostering trust and rapport. Empathy also involves putting oneself in another's shoes, considering their perspective, and offering genuine understanding and support.

Compassionate Listening

Compassionate listening forms the cornerstone of empathetic communication, enabling individuals to forge deeper connections and strengthen relationships. This practice involves being fully present in the moment, giving undivided attention to the speaker, and refraining from interruptions or distractions. Through active listening, individuals demonstrate respect and empathy, validating the experiences and emotions of others.

Moreover, compassionate listening entails empathetic responses that convey understanding and support. Reflective listening techniques, such as paraphrasing and summarizing, allow individuals to demonstrate their comprehension of the speaker's message while affirming their feelings and experiences. Additionally, asking open-ended questions encourages further exploration and fosters mutual understanding.

The qualities of kindness and empathy serve as powerful catalysts for increasing personal attractiveness and fostering meaningful connections with others. By engaging in acts of kindness, showing empathy and understanding, and practicing compassionate listening, individuals can cultivate a sense of warmth and authenticity that resonates with those around them. As we strive to navigate the complexities of human interaction, let us remember the profound impact of kindness and empathy in shaping a more compassionate and interconnected world.

Chapter 7: Developing a Positive Mindset

A positive mindset is the foundation of personal attractiveness. It involves training your mind to focus on the good in every situation, seeing challenges as opportunities for growth, and believing in your ability to overcome obstacles. Below are some ways to develop a positive mindset:

1. **Practice Self-Compassion**: Be kind to yourself, especially during difficult times. Treat yourself with the same understanding and support that you would offer to a friend facing a similar situation.

2. **Challenge Negative Thoughts**: Pay attention to your inner dialogue and challenge negative thoughts with evidence-based reasoning. Replace them with more certain and enabling convictions

3. Surrounding yourself with positivity can help reinforce a positive mindset.

4. **Focus on Solutions**: Instead of dwelling on problems, focus on finding solutions. Approach challenges with a proactive attitude and a belief that you can overcome them.

5. **Practice Mindfulness**: Mindfulness techniques, such as meditation and deep breathing exercises, can help you stay present and cultivate a positive outlook on life.

Cultivating Optimism

Optimism is the belief that good things will happen in the future, even in the face of adversity. Cultivating optimism involves adopting a hopeful attitude and reframing negative experiences in a more positive light. Here's how to cultivate optimism:

1. **Make Gratitude a habit**: Consistently offer thanks for the beneficial things in your day to day existence. Focus on what you have rather than what you lack, and you'll cultivate a more optimistic outlook.

2. **Put forth Reasonable Objectives:** Put forth feasible objectives for you and commend your advancement en route. Having a sense of purpose and direction can fuel optimism.

3. **Imagining Success**: Picture yourself accomplishing your objectives and conquering impediments. This positive visualization can help boost confidence and optimism.

4. **Learn from Failure**: Instead of viewing failure as a setback, see it as an opportunity to learn and grow. Optimistic individuals see failure as a temporary obstacle, not a permanent defeat.

5. **Surround Yourself with Optimistic People**: Spend time with people who have a hopeful outlook on life. Their positivity can be contagious and inspire you to adopt a more optimistic mindset.

Gratitude and Appreciation

Practicing gratitude and appreciation involves acknowledging the good things in your life and expressing appreciation for them. Cultivating a sense of gratitude can lead to greater happiness, improved relationships, and increased personal attractiveness. Here's how to practice gratitude and appreciation:

1. **Keep a Gratitude Journal**: Take time each day to write down three things you're

grateful for. Reflecting on the positives in your life can shift your focus away from negativity.

2. **Express Appreciation to Others**: Take the time to thank the people in your life who have supported and uplifted you. Expressing gratitude can strengthen your relationships and foster a sense of connection.

3. **Focus on the Present Moment**: Pay attention to the small moments of joy and beauty in your everyday life. Whether it's a beautiful sunset or a kind gesture from a stranger, savoring these moments can cultivate gratitude.

4. **Practice Random Acts of Kindness:** Look for opportunities to make someone else's day a little brighter. Acts of kindness not only benefit others but also increase feelings of gratitude and appreciation within yourself.

5. **Count Your Blessings**: When faced with challenges, take a moment to count your blessings and remind yourself of the good

things in your life. This perspective shift can help you maintain a sense of gratitude even during difficult times.

Resilience in the Face of Challenges

Resilience is the ability to bounce back from adversity and thrive in the face of challenges. Building resilience involves developing coping strategies, maintaining a positive outlook, and cultivating a strong support network. Here's how to build resilience:

1. **Develop Coping Strategies**: Identify healthy coping mechanisms that help you manage stress and adversity. This could include exercise, mindfulness practices, or seeking support from others.
2. **Build a Support Network**: Surround yourself with people who offer encouragement, understanding, and support during difficult times. Having a strong support network can help bolster resilience.

3. **Practice Taking care of oneself**: Focus on taking care of oneself exercises that support your physical, profound, and mental prosperity. Taking care of yourself allows you to better cope with life's challenges.

4. **Learn from Adversity**: View challenges as opportunities for growth and learning. Every setback has the potential to teach you valuable lessons that can strengthen your resilience.

5. **Maintain Perspective**: Keep things in perspective and remind yourself that setbacks are temporary. Focus on what you can control and take proactive steps to move forward.

By developing a positive mindset, cultivating optimism, practicing gratitude and appreciation, and building resilience in the face of challenges, you can increase your personal attractiveness to others. These qualities not only contribute to your own well-being but also enhance your relationships and draw others to you. Embrace these strategies, and watch as your personal magnetism grows.

Chapter 8: Building Charisma and Charm

Building Charisma and Charm

Charisma and charm are qualities that can significantly impact how others perceive and interact with us. Building charisma and charm starts from within and extends to our outward behavior and communication. Here are a few viable systems to develop these characteristics:

1. **Developing confidence**: Confidence is a key component of charisma. To fabricate certainty, center around your assets, put forth attainable objectives, and praise your victories. Practice positive self-talk and visualize yourself succeeding in various situations.

2. **Cultivating positivity**: People are naturally drawn to those with a positive attitude. Cultivate positivity by practicing gratitude, surrounding yourself with uplifting people, and reframing negative thoughts into more optimistic perspectives.

3. **Enhancing communication skills**: Effective communication is essential for charisma and charm. Practice active listening, maintain eye contact, and use open body language to convey warmth and openness. Tailor your communication style to the preferences of your audience and strive to connect with them on a personal level.

4. **Practicing empathy**: Empathy allows us to understand and relate to others' emotions and experiences. Cultivate empathy by actively listening to others, seeking to understand their perspectives, and demonstrating compassion and understanding.

5. **Refining appearance**: While physical appearance is not the sole determinant of charisma, grooming and presentation can significantly impact how others perceive us. Dressing appropriately for different occasions, maintaining good hygiene, and practicing good posture can enhance our overall presence and attractiveness.

Charismatic Communication

Charismatic communication involves engaging others through compelling storytelling, authentic expression, and effective body language. Here are some tips for enhancing your communication style:

1. **Active listening**: Show genuine interest in others by actively listening to what they have to say. Avoid interrupting and demonstrate empathy by acknowledging their thoughts and feelings.

2. **Storytelling**: Craft engaging narratives that resonate with your audience's emotions and values. Use vivid imagery, humor, and personal anecdotes to captivate their attention and convey your message effectively.

3. **Authenticity**: Communicate with sincerity and be genuine. Authenticity builds trust and rapport with others, making you more relatable and trustworthy.

4. **Body language**: Pay attention to your body language, as it can significantly impact how others perceive you. Maintain good posture, make eye contact, and use expressive gestures to convey confidence and warmth.

5. **Humor**: Appropriately timed humor can lighten the mood and foster connection with others. Use humor to break the ice, ease tension, and create a more enjoyable interaction.

Charismatic Leadership

Charismatic leaders inspire and motivate others through their vision, passion, and charisma. Here's how you can cultivate charismatic leadership qualities:

1. **Vision and purpose**: Articulate a compelling vision that inspires and motivates others to action. Communicate your vision clearly and passionately, and demonstrate commitment to achieving it.

2. **Inspirational motivation**: Motivate and energize your team members by instilling a sense of purpose and enthusiasm. Lead by example and encourage others to strive for excellence.

3. **Emotional intelligence**: Develop emotional intelligence by understanding and managing your own emotions as well as those of others. Empathize with your team members' perspectives and emotions, and respond appropriately to their needs.

4. **Building trust**: Establish trust with your team through honesty, integrity, and reliability. Keep your promises, admit mistakes, and demonstrate transparency in your actions and decisions.

5. **Empowering others**: Delegate authority and responsibility to your team members, and provide them with the support and resources they need to succeed. Encourage autonomy, innovation, and growth, and recognize and celebrate their achievements.

The Power of Charisma in Relationships

Charisma plays a crucial role in building and nurturing meaningful relationships. Here's how you can leverage charisma to enhance your relationships:

1. **Building rapport**: Connect with others on a personal level by showing genuine interest in their thoughts, feelings, and experiences. Build

rapport through active listening, empathy, and shared interests.

2. **Influence and persuasion**: Use charisma to influence and persuade others to align with your ideas or goals. Build credibility and trust, and appeal to their emotions and values to garner support for your initiatives.

3. **Conflict resolution**: Charismatic individuals are often skilled at resolving conflicts peacefully and diplomatically. Approach conflicts with an open mind, seek common ground, and communicate assertively yet empathetically to find mutually satisfactory solutions.

4. **Networking**: Charisma can be a valuable asset in networking and building professional connections. Engage others with warmth and authenticity, and seek opportunities to add value and support their goals.

5. **Building lasting connections**: Nurture your relationships over time by investing time and effort into maintaining them. Stay in touch, show appreciation for others, and be proactive in supporting their success and well-being.

cultivating charisma and charm can greatly enhance personal attractiveness and effectiveness in various aspects of life. By developing confidence, refining communication skills, embracing authenticity, and nurturing relationships, you can leverage the power of charisma to connect with others, inspire action, and achieve success.

Chapter 9: Conclusion: Embracing Personal Growth and Transformation

Embracing personal growth and transformation is an ongoing journey that can lead to increased attractiveness to others in various aspects of life. Whether it's improving physical appearance, developing emotional intelligence, honing communication skills, or cultivating a positive mindset, there are numerous avenues to explore on the path to becoming the best version of oneself.

One of the fundamental aspects of personal growth is self-awareness. This involves taking the time to reflect on one's strengths, weaknesses, values, and goals. By understanding oneself better, individuals can make more informed decisions about the areas they want to improve and the changes they want to make in their lives.

Physical attractiveness is often the first thing that comes to mind when discussing personal attractiveness. While physical appearance can play a role in how others perceive us, true attractiveness goes beyond outward appearances. It encompasses confidence, charisma, and a sense of authenticity. However, taking care of one's physical health and appearance can boost self-confidence and contribute to overall well-being.

Exercise, proper nutrition, and adequate rest are essential components of maintaining physical health. Regular physical activity not only improves physical fitness but also releases endorphins, which can enhance mood and reduce stress. Eating a balanced diet rich in fruits, vegetables, lean proteins, and whole grains provides the body with the nutrients it needs to function optimally.

In addition to physical health, emotional intelligence is crucial for personal growth and attractiveness. Emotional intelligence encompasses the ability to recognize, understand, and manage both our own emotions and the emotions of others. Individuals with high emotional intelligence are often perceived as empathetic, resilient, and socially adept.

Developing emotional intelligence involves practices such as self-reflection, active listening, and empathy. By cultivating these skills, individuals can build stronger interpersonal relationships, navigate conflicts more effectively, and demonstrate greater emotional stability.

Communication skills are another essential aspect of personal growth and attractiveness.Powerful correspondence includes putting oneself out there obviously as well as listening effectively and compassionately. It's about conveying ideas, thoughts, and feelings in a way that fosters understanding and connection with others.

Improving communication skills can involve techniques such as assertiveness training, public speaking practice, and conflict resolution strategies. By becoming better communicators, individuals can enhance their personal and professional relationships, build trust, and influence others positively.

A positive mindset is a powerful tool for personal growth and attractiveness. Maintaining a positive outlook can help individuals overcome challenges, bounce back from setbacks, and approach life with resilience and optimism. Cultivating gratitude, practicing mindfulness, and reframing negative thoughts are all ways to foster a positive mindset.

Self-care is an integral part of personal growth and transformation. It involves prioritizing one's physical, emotional, and mental well-being through activities that nourish and rejuvenate the body and mind. Self-care practices can vary widely from person to person and may include exercise, meditation, hobbies, spending time with loved ones, or simply taking time to relax and unwind.

Ultimately, embracing personal growth and transformation is about investing in oneself and committing to continual improvement. It's about recognizing that change is possible and taking proactive steps to become the best version of oneself. By focusing on self-awareness, physical health, emotional intelligence, communication skills, positive mindset, and self-care, individuals can increase their personal attractiveness to others and create a more fulfilling and meaningful life.